MIA STONE

TOP 20 HOME WORKOUTS FOR WOMEN

Lose Weight, Sculpt, and Tone - No Gym Required!

This book was professionally typeset on Reedsy.
Find out more at reedsy.com

Contents

Introduction

Welcome to a fresh start, a practical, no-nonsense approach to getting fit and feeling fabulous—all from the comfort of your own home. If you're reading this, you're probably on the lookout for effective workouts that don't require endless hours, a gym membership, or expensive equipment. Maybe you're juggling work, family, and personal commitments, with just enough time left for a quick cup of coffee, let alone a full workout session. Sound familiar? If so, you're exactly who this book was written for.

As someone who's been down the same road, I know firsthand the struggles of finding the time, motivation, and right workouts to achieve the results you want. I wrote this book to take the guesswork out of your fitness routine and to empower you with the tools you need to achieve your goals without needing anything more than some basic equipment and a commitment to your health. Through research, testing, and years of experience, I've crafted a guide that's efficient, accessible, and, most importantly, effective.

This isn't about crash diets or impossible fitness routines that leave you burned out. Instead, it's about real workouts designed for real women, who want results. Whether you want to lose weight, sculpt your body, or tone up, every workout in this book has been created to target these goals in simple, achievable steps. You'll find routines for your lower body, upper body, core, and even a few cardio blasters that will keep your heart rate up, your calories burning, and your body steadily transforming. I've also added some quick 20-minute routines to keep things manageable even on your busiest days and wrap up with a 28-day weight loss challenge to get you seeing results right away.

Here's a sneak peek at what's coming your way. First, we'll start with the basics—the foundation of what makes a workout effective and how to do it safely at home. Next, we'll walk through goal setting to help you focus on what you want to achieve and understand what your body needs to get there. Injury prevention is also key; I'll share tips to help you nail your form and keep your joints happy while working out solo. After that, it's all about getting into the workouts: chapters dedicated to sculpting and strengthening your lower body, upper body, and core. Each section will feature exercises carefully chosen for maximum impact, allowing you to work on each area of your body in the most time-efficient way possible, but keeping it fun (after all, if it isn't fun, what's the point, right)?

When time is tight, I've got you covered with quick and effective 20-minute workouts that you can rotate throughout the week. Finally, my 28-day challenge will guide you day by day, keeping you on track toward your goals with a structured plan that makes it easy to stay motivated and track your progress.

This book is designed to be your go-to guide whenever you want to squeeze in a workout, no matter where you are in your fitness journey. So, get ready to jump in, feel strong, and start seeing the results you've been dreaming of. Let's kick things off by understanding the foundations of effective home workouts in the next chapter.

Chapter 2: Foundations of Home Workouts

Working out at home is more than just an alternative to the gym—it's a powerful way to prioritize your health while fitting seamlessly into your lifestyle. If you're like many women balancing a full schedule, myself included, the thought of hitting the gym can feel like just another commitment to juggle. But home workouts bring fitness to you, no commute, no crowded locker rooms, and no waiting around for equipment. This chapter lays out the unique advantages of home workouts, making it easier to see why this approach works so well for busy schedules and unique fitness needs.

Convenience

One of the biggest benefits of home workouts is how seamlessly they fit into even the busiest schedules. When you're working out at home, there's no need to carve out extra time for commuting to and from a gym. Instead, you can transition from your day right into a workout with ease, whether that's right after breakfast, during a quick lunch break, or in the evening when things settle down. This flexibility allows you to focus on what really matters—your fitness—without the hassle of traveling or waiting for equipment to free up.

With a home workout routine, you're in control of your time. You don't have to work around gym hours or worry about crowded peak times; you can simply pick up your mat and start moving whenever it suits you best. This freedom to exercise on your own schedule makes it much easier to stay consistent. Whether you have a full hour or just 20 minutes, there's always an opportunity to fit in some movement. You're creating a routine that's tailored to your life and priorities, making it easier to stay on track and see real results.

Cost-Effectiveness

One of the most appealing aspects of home workouts is how budget-friendly they can be. Gym memberships, classes, and personal training sessions can add up quickly, but with a home workout routine, you get the freedom to focus on fitness without the ongoing expense. This book is designed with that in mind—everything here is geared toward helping you maximize results without needing to invest in expensive gym equipment or pay recurring fees.

The exercises in this book rely primarily on your own body weight, making it easy to jump into each workout with minimal setup. Body weight exercises, like squats, lunges, and planks, are incredibly effective for building strength, burning calories, and improving endurance. If you want to add a little extra resistance, basic items like a set of resistance bands or a couple of dumbbells can give you plenty of options without breaking the bank (but they are totally optional). This simplicity allows you to focus on what truly matters—your health and progress—while keeping your workout routine accessible and affordable.

Flexibility in Routine

One of the most empowering aspects of home workouts is the freedom to design a routine that's uniquely yours. Unlike the structured environment of a gym or class, where you might feel pressured to follow a set format or keep up with others, working out at home allows you to customize each session to suit your needs, preferences, and fitness level. This book provides a variety of workouts and exercises to help you mix and match, so you can create a plan that fits perfectly with your goals—whether that's weight loss, muscle toning, or simply staying active.

When you're working out at home, you can adjust the intensity, type, and duration of your workouts based on what feels right for you on any given day. Maybe you're in the mood for a quick, intense session to get your heart pumping, or perhaps you'd rather spend a bit more time focusing on strength and technique. This flexibility not only keeps your routine interesting, but also makes it easier to stay consistent, as you're no longer limited by the constraints of a class schedule or equipment availability. Working out at home allows you to prioritize what works best for you, creating a fitness routine that's as adaptable as it is effective.

Personal Environment

One of the greatest advantages of working out at home is the freedom to create a personal space that feels inviting and comfortable, free from the pressures that often come with a gym environment. For many, walking into a gym—especially when just starting a fitness journey—can feel intimidating. The crowded equipment, unfamiliar machines, and often competitive atmosphere can make it difficult to feel at ease. But at home, you're in full control, and that freedom can make all the difference in building a positive workout experience.

In your personal space, you can set the tone exactly how you want.

Whether it's blasting your favorite music (and singing along of course), wearing what feels most comfortable (we can't always be in our cutest workout clothes), or moving at your own pace, working out at home allows you to create an environment that motivates you without any external pressure. This sense of comfort and privacy is especially valuable for beginners, giving you a chance to build confidence in your own space. As you progress, the ability to work out in a setting that feels completely your own becomes a powerful tool in making fitness a sustainable part of your life. Now that we know a little bit about the foundations of working out at home, let's understand more about your fitness goals in the next chapter.

Chapter 3: Setting Your Fitness Goals

Setting fitness goals is about more than simply deciding to exercise; it's about creating a clear path toward the health and strength you envision. Goals give you purpose and focus, providing the motivation needed to stay consistent, even when things get challenging (holiday season anyone). This chapter is designed to help you set practical, actionable goals that align with your lifestyle and keep you inspired along the way. Whether you're aiming to lose weight, build strength, or increase endurance, having well-defined goals will transform your fitness journey into a rewarding and sustainable experience.

The Importance of Goal-Setting

Setting clear fitness goals is like creating a roadmap for your workout journey. Without defined goals, it's easy to feel aimless, wondering if the time and effort you're putting in are actually making a difference. By establishing specific fitness goals, you give your routine direction and purpose, zeroing in on what you truly want to achieve—whether it's weight loss, increased strength, or better endurance. Goals help you prioritize your workouts, turning each session into a step toward measurable progress.

When you set goals, you also gain a powerful tool for tracking that progress. Having concrete benchmarks allows you to see if you're on track, which can be incredibly motivating and help keep your efforts consistent. Instead of guessing, you'll have measurable data, whether it's tracking how many reps you can do, noting weight loss, or observing improvements in stamina. This insight helps you adjust your approach as needed, making sure that every minute you spend working out is moving you closer to the results you want. Goal-setting isn't just about reaching a finish line; it's about making your fitness journey purposeful and rewarding every step of the way.

Identify Personal Motivations

Setting goals is essential, but understanding the "why" behind those goals is what truly fuels your fitness journey. Digging deep to uncover your personal motivations can make all the difference when it comes to staying consistent and committed. Why do you want to start this journey? What do you hope to gain from it? For some, it might be the desire to feel stronger and more empowered in their own body. For others, it could be about building confidence, boosting self-esteem, or having more energy to keep up with family and life's demands.

These personal motivations are more than just ideas—they're the heart of your journey. When you're feeling tired or tempted to skip a workout, reminding yourself of these "whys" can reignite your determination. Maybe you want to set a positive example for your kids, or perhaps you're looking to reclaim a sense of control and well-being in your life. Whatever your reasons, they're uniquely yours and powerful enough to drive real change. Keep them close and revisit them often; they're the key to transforming your fitness goals into something meaningful and lasting.

Track Progress Efficiently

Tracking your progress is one of the most effective ways to stay motivated and ensure you're on the right path. When you take the time to log your workouts, note changes, and celebrate milestones, you're creating a visual record of your hard work—a reminder that each session is moving you closer to your goals. Progress tracking doesn't need to be complicated; it can be as simple as keeping a journal, marking workout days on a calendar, or using a fitness app. These small actions make it easier to see patterns, recognize areas for improvement, and stay consistent.

Tracking also gives you the data needed to adjust your approach as you go. Maybe you notice that you're doing more reps than when you started, or you're completing cardio sessions with more ease. These indicators of progress are essential for keeping you engaged and focused on the big picture, even when day-to-day changes might be subtle. Over time, tracking progress turns into a powerful motivation tool, proving that every effort you put in is adding up. Celebrate each win, big or small—they're all signs of growth that keep you energized and committed. Ok, now that we've learned more about the importance of goal setting, let's dive into the basics of your body and its primary muscle groups in the next chapter.

Chapter 4: Understanding Your Body: The Basics

Getting the most out of your workouts isn't just about going through the motions; it's about understanding the muscles you're working and why each movement matters. This chapter provides a simple, clear overview of the primary muscle groups and how they function, helping you connect each exercise to its target area. When you know which muscles you're working, you gain better control over your body and make each movement more effective. Understanding the basics of your body not only makes your workouts more rewarding, but also sets a strong foundation for balanced and sustainable fitness.

Introduction to the Four Major Muscle Groups

When it comes to working out, focusing on the body's primary muscle groups—arms, legs, core, and back—can make a huge difference in building strength, balance, and overall fitness. These four muscle groups support nearly every movement we make, from everyday tasks to more intense exercises, and when toned, they're key to achieving a fit, lean, and strong appearance. Understanding what each group does can help you approach workouts with purpose, making each exercise count.

Arms: Your arms are responsible for many upper-body movements, including lifting, pushing, and pulling. Key muscles here include the biceps and triceps, which work together to move and stabilize your arms. Strengthening these muscles not only helps with functional movements—like carrying groceries or lifting a child—but also shapes your arms, giving them a defined, toned look. Exercises that target the arms can give you that sculpted, fit appearance that's both strong and feminine.

Legs: The muscles in your legs, including the quadriceps, hamstrings, and calves, are some of the strongest in the body. These muscles help with stability, mobility, and power, making them essential for movements like walking, running, squatting, and jumping. Working on leg strength builds a solid foundation for the rest of your body, allowing you to move more efficiently and with greater endurance. When toned, they add shape and definition to your thighs and calves, giving your legs a sleek and athletic look that reflects all your hard work.

Core: Often referred to as the body's "powerhouse," the core includes muscles around the abdomen, lower back, and sides. A strong core stabilizes your spine, improves posture, and supports balance. Every time you perform an exercise—whether it's lifting weights or stretching—your core muscles are working to keep you steady. Toning your core not only supports physical activities and reduces strain on your back, but also helps flatten and tighten your midsection, creating that lean, strong look many of us strive for.

Back: The back muscles, including the lats (latissimus dorsi) and traps (trapezius), support posture, allow for pulling movements, and play a key role in upper body strength. A strong back is essential for exercises like rows and pull-ups, and it helps maintain a balanced body, reducing the risk of slouching or back pain. Focusing on these muscles ensures you're building a strong, well-rounded upper body, and it can also add a toned, defined look to your back and shoulders, helping you achieve a balanced, athletic appearance that's visible from all angles.

Each of these four muscle groups contributes to a balanced and effective workout routine and, when toned, creates a body that looks and feels fit. By understanding how they work together, you can design workouts that target these areas in a way that enhances both your body's strength and appearance, supporting your fitness goals and giving you that strong, confident look.

Link Exercises to Muscle Groups

Knowing which exercises target specific muscle groups can transform your workout, allowing you to focus on the areas you want to strengthen and tone. When you understand the connection between exercises and muscle groups, you're able to select workouts that deliver the results you're looking for, whether it's shaping your arms, sculpting your legs, tightening your core, or strengthening your back.

For instance, if your goal is to work on your arms, exercises like push-ups, and tricep dips are highly effective. Push-ups engage not only the biceps and triceps, but also the shoulders, giving your upper body a well-rounded workout (this is why it is one of the best exercises for shredding your upper body in a short amount of time). These exercises help add tone and definition to your arms, creating a sculpted look.

When it comes to shaping and strengthening your legs, exercises like squats, lunges, and glute bridges are perfect choices. Squats and lunges focus on the quads, hamstrings, and glutes, providing a complete lower-body workout that helps to define and firm your legs, giving them an athletic, toned appearance. Glute bridges, meanwhile, target the glutes specifically, adding shape and definition to your bum.

For your core, exercises such as planks, crunches, and bicycle twists are excellent for building strength and stability. These moves focus on the abdominals and obliques, helping you achieve a flatter, more toned midsection. Core exercises are particularly important because they not only improve appearance, but also enhance balance and protect the lower back.

Finally, back-focused exercises pushups work the latissimus dorsi, trapezius, and other upper back muscles. These exercises strengthen the back and shoulders, helping to improve posture and add a toned, defined look to your upper body. A strong back also balances out your upper body's appearance, complementing the work you put into your arms and core.

By linking exercises to the muscle groups you want to target, you're able to design a workout that focuses on specific areas while still supporting full-body balance. This approach makes your routine more purposeful, helping you achieve a toned, well-proportioned look across all major muscle groups.

Importance of Muscle Balance

Muscle balance is essential for building strength safely and effectively. When you work out, it's tempting to focus on the areas you want to tone or strengthen the most, but giving attention to all muscle groups—especially those that work in pairs or opposites—keeps your body balanced and reduces the risk of injury. Muscle imbalances occur when one muscle group becomes significantly stronger than its counterpart, leading to strain on joints and potential discomfort over time.

For example, if you consistently focus on exercises that build the chest and neglect the upper back, it can lead to poor posture and tightness in the shoulders. Similarly, overdeveloping the quadriceps without paying attention to the hamstrings can put extra stress on your knees, increasing the likelihood of injury. By working both sides of these muscle pairs—like chest and back, or quads and hamstrings—you ensure that your body stays strong and aligned.

Balanced muscles also enhance overall performance, making you more stable and efficient in all movements, both in workouts and in daily activities. Strengthening each muscle group evenly provides a solid foundation, allowing your body to move with ease and preventing overuse injuries. A balanced workout approach, like the one outlined in this book, helps you achieve a body that not only looks fit, but also feels strong and resilient.

Benefits of Muscle Awareness

Muscle awareness, or the ability to connect your mind to the muscles you're working, is a powerful tool in achieving more effective workouts. When you have a strong mind-body connection, you're able to feel and control each movement with precision, focusing on the muscles being engaged. This heightened awareness not only makes exercises more effective, but also helps improve form, prevent injury, and make every rep count.

When you truly focus on the muscles you're using—whether it's your core during a plank, your glutes in a squat, or your back in a pushup—

you activate them more fully, maximizing their potential with each movement. This engagement helps you work out with intention, so you're not just going through the motions, but actively challenging and strengthening your body.

Muscle awareness also allows you to adjust and refine your form, ensuring that each exercise is done safely and correctly. As you become more in tune with your body, you can better recognize when an exercise feels right or if something is off, which can prevent common mistakes that lead to strain or injury. This connection ultimately enhances the quality of your workouts, making them not only more effective, but also more enjoyable. As you build muscle awareness, you'll feel more empowered and confident, fully engaged in each workout and aware of the progress your body is making. Ok, now that we know more about our muscles, let's learn a little bit about how to prevent injury to them while working out at home in the next chapter.

Chapter 5: Injury Prevention at Home: Focus on Form and Safety

Preventing injuries is a crucial part of any workout routine, and when you're exercising at home, it becomes even more important. Without a trainer by your side to correct your form, focusing on technique and safety is essential to avoid strains, sprains, and other common injuries. This chapter will guide you through the key practices that can help you stay safe, so you can confidently get the most out of your workouts. By taking a few extra steps to warm up, cool down, and listen to your body, you'll create a safe, sustainable routine that keeps you moving toward your goals without setbacks.

Warm-Up and Cool-Down Routines

Starting each workout with a proper warm-up and ending with a cool-down is one of the simplest and most effective ways to prevent injuries. A warm-up gently prepares your muscles, joints, and cardiovascular system for the exercises ahead. By increasing blood flow to your muscles and gradually raising your heart rate, you're priming your body to handle more intense movements safely and efficiently. Warm-ups also help loosen any tightness, which can reduce the risk of strains or sprains during your workout. Just a few minutes of light cardio, dynamic stretching, or controlled movements like arm circles or leg swings is enough to wake up your body and get it ready to move.

Cooling down is equally important and often overlooked. After a workout, your muscles are warm and have been under strain, so gradually easing them back into rest mode is essential. A cool-down helps lower your heart rate slowly, preventing dizziness or lightheadedness, and allows your muscles to relax and lengthen. Simple stretches targeting the muscles you've worked—like hamstring stretches after leg exercises or gentle twists after core work—help release any tightness and improve flexibility. Cooling down not only aids in muscle recovery, reducing soreness, but also prepares your body for your next workout. A few minutes of intentional warm-up and cool-down can be the key to maintaining a safe and sustainable fitness routine.

Listen to Your Body

Listening to your body is one of the most crucial aspects of injury prevention and long-term fitness success. Too often, people push themselves beyond their current capabilities, driven by the desire to progress faster or match what others are doing. While challenging yourself is an important part of growth, there's a fine line between pushing your limits and risking injury. Learning to recognize the difference between healthy discomfort and actual pain is key to knowing when to keep going and when to pause (slow and steady wins the race).

Discomfort, like the burn you feel during the last few reps or the effort required to maintain a plank, is normal and expected. It signals that your muscles are working and adapting. Pain, on the other hand, is your body's way of alerting you that something isn't right—whether it's a sharp twinge, a sudden ache, or a feeling of strain in a joint or tendon. Ignoring these signals can lead to overuse injuries or strains that could sideline you from your goals.

Listening to your body also means giving yourself permission to rest and recover. Rest days are essential for muscle repair and growth, and they help prevent burnout. If an exercise feels too challenging or uncomfortable, try a modified version or take a break. There's no rush to master every movement right away; gradual, mindful progress ensures you're building strength safely and sustainably. By tuning into your body's signals, you'll develop a workout routine that respects your limits while helping you reach your fitness goals without unnecessary setbacks.

Education on Common Injuries and Prevention

Understanding common fitness injuries and how to prevent them is essential for maintaining a safe and effective workout routine. Knees, lower back, and shoulders are particularly vulnerable areas during workouts, especially in exercises like squats, lunges, and core work where alignment and form are key. By being mindful of proper technique, you can greatly reduce the risk of strain or injury to these sensitive areas.

Knees: Knee injuries are often caused by poor alignment during exercises like squats and lunges. To protect your knees, ensure that they stay aligned over your ankles, rather than collapsing inward or jutting too far forward. During squats, keep your weight evenly distributed through your feet, engaging your glutes and core to support the movement. When performing lunges, aim for a 90-degree angle in both knees, with your front knee directly above your ankle. These small adjustments can relieve excess pressure on the knee joints, keeping them safe and strong.

Lower Back: The lower back is susceptible to strain, particularly in core exercises and weight-bearing movements. To avoid lower back injuries, focus on engaging your core and maintaining a neutral spine throughout each movement. In exercises like planks, avoid letting your hips sag or rise too high, as this can put undue pressure on the lower back.

Shoulders: Shoulder injuries are common, especially when performing exercises that involve the upper body. To protect your shoulders, avoid overextending or straining the shoulder joint. Keep your shoulders down and back, avoiding "shrugging" them up towards your ears, which can lead to tension and strain. For exercises like push-ups or shoulder presses, maintain a stable shoulder position, and ensure that your arms are moving in a controlled, natural range of motion.

By paying close attention to alignment and proper technique, you can protect these common injury-prone areas and strengthen your body in a balanced way. Practicing good form not only reduces the risk of injury, but also makes each movement more effective, allowing you to get the most out of your workouts safely. A little extra focus on alignment and awareness goes a long way toward building a sustainable and injury-free fitness routine. Now that we've delved into the importance of injury prevention, let's dive into some exercises. In the next chapter, we're going to learn all about the powerhouse exercise of your legs, the squat.

Chapter 6: Lower Body Sculpting

Sculpting and toning the lower body is one of the most rewarding parts of any fitness routine. Strong, toned legs and glutes not only enhance your figure, but also improve stability, balance, and endurance. This chapter dives into some of the most effective exercises for the lower body—squats, lunges, glute bridges, and side leg lifts—each offering a range of techniques and variations to keep your workouts challenging and adaptable to your fitness level. With a focus on proper form and progression, these exercises will help you build strength and definition in your legs, thighs, and glutes, creating a strong and sculpted lower body.

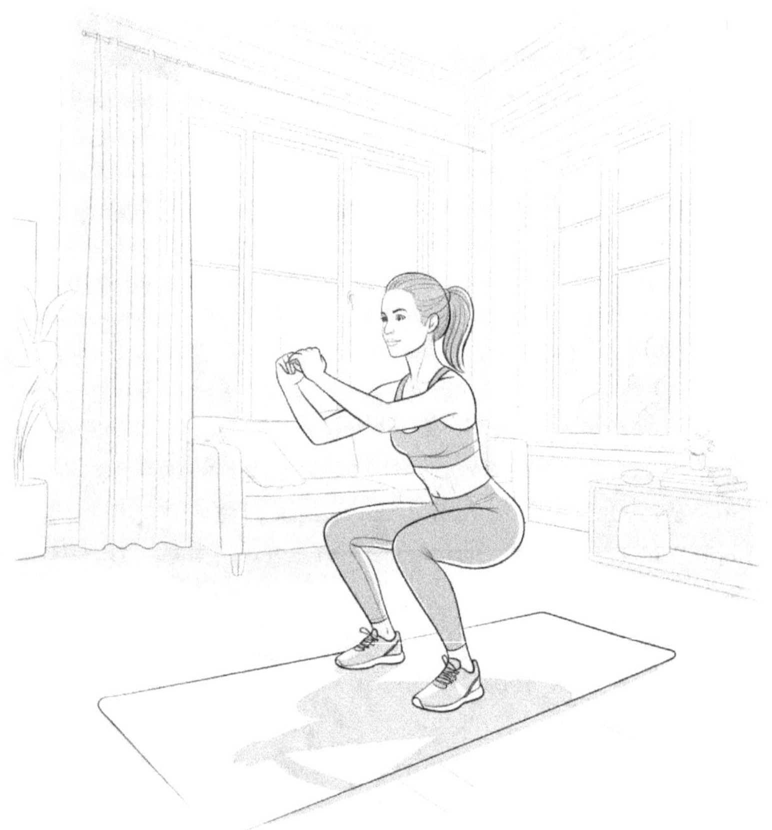

Basic Squat Form

The squat is a foundational exercise for lower body strength and toning, targeting key muscles like the quadriceps, hamstrings, glutes, and core. Here's how to perform a basic squat:

Starting Position:

- Stand with your feet about hip-width apart.
- Point your toes slightly outward for balance and stability.
- Engage your core by pulling your belly button toward your spine

to support your lower back.

Movement:

- Begin by bending at the hips and knees, as if sitting back into a chair.
- Keep your chest lifted and shoulders back throughout the movement.
- Distribute your weight evenly in your feet, pressing through your heels.
- Lower yourself until your thighs are parallel to the floor or as low as comfortable.
- Ensure your knees stay aligned with your toes to avoid strain.

Returning to Standing:

- Press through your heels to rise back to a standing position.
- Engage your glutes as you come up for added strength and toning.

Practicing proper squat form helps you target the right muscles while minimizing injury risk. With consistency, the basic squat builds a strong foundation for more advanced movements, enhancing both strength and muscle tone in the lower body.

Squat Variations

Adding variations to your basic squat helps target different muscles in the lower body and keeps your workout interesting. Here are three popular squat variations to try, each with unique benefits for toning and strengthening your legs, glutes, and inner thighs.

Sumo Squat:

- **How to Do It**: Stand with your feet wider than hip-width apart and turn your toes out at about a 45-degree angle. Lower into a squat by bending at the knees and hips, keeping your chest lifted. Press through your heels to return to standing.
- **Muscles Targeted**: The wide stance places extra emphasis on the inner thighs and glutes, making this variation ideal for shaping and toning the inner leg muscles while still working the quads and hamstrings.

Pulse Squat:

- **How to Do It**: Start in a standard squat position, lowering yourself until your thighs are parallel to the floor. Instead of standing back up, make small up-and-down movements, or "pulses," within a few inches of your lowest squat position.
- **Muscles Targeted**: The pulse squat keeps your muscles under continuous tension, especially targeting the quads and glutes. This variation enhances muscle endurance and increases burn, helping to build a more defined lower body.

Plie Squat:

- **How to Do It**: Stand with your feet wider than shoulder-width apart, with toes pointed outwards at a 45-degree angle. Lower down by bending your knees and keeping your torso upright, similar to a ballet plie. Press through your heels to stand back up.
- **Muscles Targeted**: The plie squat focuses heavily on the inner

thighs and glutes, while also working the quads and calves. This variation is great for toning the inner thighs and enhancing flexibility in the hips.

Each squat variation adds a new challenge and targets your muscles from different angles, allowing you to achieve balanced strength and tone throughout your lower body. Integrating these variations into your routine provides variety and depth to your workouts.

Squat Modifications for Various Fitness Levels

Squats are versatile and can be adjusted to suit any fitness level, whether you're a beginner just getting started or looking to increase the challenge as you progress. Here are some modifications to help you get the most out of your squats, no matter your current level.

Wall Squat (Beginner):

- **How to Do It**: Stand with your back against a wall, feet hip-width apart, and about a foot away from the wall. Slowly lower yourself down the wall until your thighs are parallel to the floor, keeping your back supported against the wall. Hold briefly, then push through your heels to return to standing.
- **Benefits**: This modification provides extra support, helping beginners learn the squat movement while building strength and balance.

Chair-Assisted Squat (Beginner/Intermediate):

- **How to Do It**: Stand in front of a sturdy chair with your feet hip-width apart. Lower into a squat until you're just about to sit on the chair, then push through your heels to stand back up.

- **Benefits**: Using a chair helps with control and ensures you're not going too low. It's an excellent way to practice form and build confidence.

Shallow Squat (Beginner):

- **How to Do It**: Perform a squat, but only go down halfway instead of reaching a full squat depth. Focus on keeping your form and balance as you lower and raise back up.
- **Benefits**: This variation allows beginners to get comfortable with the squat movement while strengthening their lower body without putting strain on the knees.

Weighted Squat (Intermediate/Advanced):

- **How to Do It**: Hold a pair of dumbbells at your shoulders or a kettlebell at chest level as you perform a squat. Lower down as usual, then press through your heels to stand back up.
- **Benefits**: Adding weights increases resistance, making the squat more challenging and helping build strength in the legs, glutes, and core.

Deep Squat (Advanced):

- **How to Do It**: Perform a squat, but lower yourself deeper than parallel, aiming to go as low as is comfortable while maintaining good form. Keep your core tight and press through your heels to return to standing.
- **Benefits**: Going deeper engages more muscle fibers in the glutes and quads, adding intensity and improving flexibility and range of

motion in the hips.

These squat modifications allow you to progress safely, adapting to your body's needs and fitness level. By starting with the basics and gradually increasing the difficulty, you can enjoy the benefits of squats without risking injury, building strength and tone at your own pace.

Benefits of Squats

Squats are one of the most effective exercises for building lower body strength and achieving a toned, sculpted appearance. This simple movement offers a wide range of benefits that go beyond aesthetics, making it a must-have in any fitness routine. Here's why squats are so beneficial:

- **Strengthen Multiple Muscle Groups**: Squats target key muscle groups in the lower body, including the quadriceps, hamstrings, glutes, and calves, as well as the core. By working these muscles together, squats help build balanced strength that supports both fitness and daily movement.
- **Enhance Functional Fitness**: The movement pattern of squatting mimics everyday actions, like sitting, bending, and lifting. Practicing squats regularly improves your ability to perform these movements with ease and reduces the risk of strain or injury in daily life.
- **Boost Calorie Burn**: Squats engage large muscle groups, which increases the number of calories burned during and after your workout. This makes squats an efficient exercise for those looking to support weight loss and build lean muscle.
- **Improve Balance and Stability**: Squats challenge your core and lower body stability, improving your balance and coordination over time. A strong lower body and core enhance overall body control,

making you more stable in other exercises and daily activities.

- **Increase Joint Flexibility and Mobility**: Performing squats through a full range of motion helps improve flexibility in the hips, knees, and ankles. Better joint mobility not only enhances your squat form, but also supports a greater range of movement in other exercises.

- **Support Bone and Joint Health**: Weight-bearing exercises like squats stimulate bone density and strengthen the tendons and ligaments around your joints. This can help reduce the risk of osteoporosis and maintain joint health as you age.

Incorporating squats into your routine is a powerful way to achieve weight loss goals while toning and shaping the lower body. By activating major muscle groups, burning calories, and sculpting the legs and glutes, squats help you create a leaner, fitter version of yourself. Whether your aim is weight loss, improved muscle tone, or a more defined lower body, squats deliver a range of results that keep you looking and feeling your best.

Basic Lunge Form

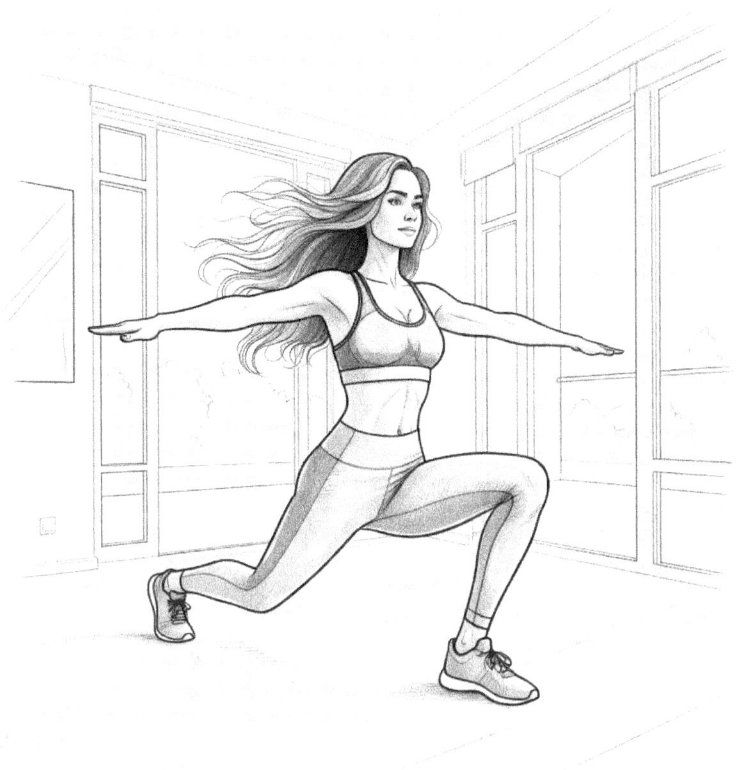

The lunge is a fundamental lower body exercise that builds strength and definition in the legs and glutes while also improving balance and coordination. Performing a basic lunge correctly ensures you're targeting the right muscles and setting a solid foundation for more advanced movements.

Starting Position:

- Stand upright with your feet together, hands resting on your hips or by your sides for balance.
- Engage your core to maintain stability throughout the movement.

Movement:

- Step one foot forward, keeping your torso upright and your shoulders stacked over your hips.
- As you step forward, lower your back knee toward the floor, aiming for a 90-degree angle in both knees. Your front knee should be aligned directly above your ankle, not extending past your toes.
- Keep your weight centered and focus on pressing through the heel of your front foot to engage the glutes and quads.

Returning to Standing:

- Push through your front heel to rise back up, bringing your front foot back to meet your other foot and returning to the starting position.
- Repeat on the opposite leg to complete one full repetition.

Practicing proper lunge form helps you strengthen and tone the muscles in your thighs, glutes, and calves while also enhancing balance. The lunge is a versatile exercise that, when done correctly, contributes to a lean, sculpted lower body and a stable foundation for various movements.

Lunge Variations

Adding lunge variations to your routine helps target different muscles in the lower body and keeps your workouts dynamic and challenging. Each variation works the legs, glutes, and core from a different angle, allowing for balanced toning and sculpting of the lower body. Here are some effective lunge variations and the muscles they target:

Reverse Lunge:

- **How to Do It**: Start in a standing position and step one foot back, lowering your back knee toward the floor while keeping your front knee aligned over your ankle. Press through the heel of your front foot to return to standing.
- **Muscles Targeted**: The reverse lunge places greater emphasis on the glutes and hamstrings, helping to tone and lift the backside while also strengthening the quads and core.

Side Lunge:

- **How to Do It**: Stand with your feet together, then step one foot out to the side. Bend the knee of the stepping leg, keeping the opposite leg straight, and lower your body toward the floor while keeping your chest lifted. Push through the heel of your bent leg to return to standing.
- **Muscles Targeted**: Side lunges work the inner thighs and outer glutes, providing a unique stretch and strengthening effect for the hips. This variation is ideal for toning the inner thighs and building lateral strength.

Walking Lunge:

- **How to Do It**: Begin with a basic forward lunge, stepping forward with one leg and lowering into the lunge position. Instead of stepping back to the starting position, step forward with the opposite leg, moving continuously as you alternate lunges with each step.
- **Muscles Targeted**: Walking lunges engage the quads, glutes, and hamstrings, while also challenging balance and coordination. This

dynamic movement helps improve endurance, muscle tone, and cardiovascular fitness, making it a great option for sculpting the legs and boosting calorie burn.

Curtsy Lunge:

- **How to Do It**: Stand with your feet together, then step one leg back and diagonally behind the other leg, lowering into a lunge. Keep your front knee aligned with your toes and your chest upright. Press through your front heel to return to standing, then switch sides.
- **Muscles Targeted**: The curtsy lunge targets the glutes, especially the outer glutes, and engages the inner thighs. This variation is perfect for shaping the hip area and building balance, giving a rounded and sculpted look to the lower body.

Incorporating these lunge variations allows you to target specific muscle groups from different angles, creating a balanced and well-defined lower body. These variations add variety to your workouts, helping you progress and prevent plateaus while building strength and tone throughout the legs and glutes.

Lunge Modifications for Various Fitness Levels

Lunges are versatile and can be adjusted to meet different fitness levels, making them accessible and effective for everyone. Here are some modifications to help you get the most out of lunges, no matter your experience or strength level.

Stationary Lunge (Beginner):

- **How to Do It**: Instead of stepping forward or backward, keep your feet in place as you lower into the lunge, focusing on form and stability. Stand with one foot in front of the other, lower down into a lunge, and then push back up without moving your feet.
- **Benefits**: The stationary lunge eliminates the need for balance while stepping, helping beginners build leg strength and perfect their form in a controlled way.

Assisted Lunge (Beginner):

- **How to Do It**: Use a chair, wall, or sturdy surface for support. Place one hand on the support as you perform a forward or reverse lunge to help with balance and control.
- **Benefits**: Assistance provides extra stability, allowing beginners to focus on the lunge movement without worrying about balance, which is especially helpful when just starting out.

Shallow Lunge (Beginner):

- **How to Do It**: Perform a lunge, but only lower yourself halfway, rather than going into a full range of motion. Focus on keeping your core engaged and your front knee aligned over your ankle.
- **Benefits**: This modification reduces the intensity on the knees and helps build confidence and strength gradually, making lunges more accessible for those who are still building lower body strength.

Weighted Lunge (Intermediate/Advanced):

- **How to Do It**: Hold a pair of dumbbells by your sides or a single dumbbell at chest level while performing a lunge. Keep your upper body stable and focus on moving with control.

- **Benefits**: Adding weights increases resistance, which challenges the quads, hamstrings, and glutes further. This modification is ideal for those looking to increase muscle tone and build strength.

Walking Lunge with Twist (Advanced):

- **How to Do It**: Perform a walking lunge, but add a twist by rotating your torso toward your front leg at the bottom of each lunge. Use a light weight or medicine ball for an added challenge.
- **Benefits**: The twist engages the core, increasing stability and strength, while the walking motion boosts endurance and calorie burn. This advanced modification is excellent for improving balance and coordination.

Elevated Lunge (Advanced):

- **How to Do It**: Place your back foot on a stable surface, like a bench or step, and perform a lunge with your front leg. This modification, often called a Bulgarian split squat, requires more balance and leg strength.
- **Benefits**: The elevated lunge increases the intensity on the front leg, providing a deeper stretch for the glutes and quads, and helps develop single-leg strength and balance.

These lunge modifications allow you to scale the intensity of your workouts to match your fitness level, helping you build strength, tone, and endurance progressively. By choosing the right variation, you can enjoy the benefits of lunges without over straining, making this essential exercise accessible and challenging at every stage of your fitness journey.

Benefits of Lunges

Lunges are a highly effective lower body exercise that offers a range of benefits for strength, toning, and functional fitness. This versatile movement targets multiple muscles, improving balance, coordination, and overall body alignment. Here's why lunges are such a valuable addition to any workout routine:

- **Tones and Sculpts Legs and Glutes**: Lunges are excellent for targeting the quadriceps, hamstrings, and glutes, making them ideal for shaping and toning the thighs and backside. Consistently performing lunges helps define and strengthen the legs, creating a lean, sculpted appearance.
- **Promotes Balance and Stability**: Since lunges work one leg at a time, they challenge your balance and engage the core to keep you stable. This unilateral movement helps improve coordination, making you more stable in everyday movements and supporting better posture.
- **Builds Functional Strength**: Lunges mimic natural movements, like stepping forward or bending down, which improves your ability to perform everyday tasks. Building strength through lunges helps you move with more ease and reduces the risk of strains in real-life activities, like climbing stairs or picking up objects.
- **Enhances Calorie Burn and Supports Weight Loss**: Lunges engage large muscle groups, which requires more energy and increases calorie burn. This makes lunges a great exercise for those looking to support weight loss goals while building lean muscle in the lower body.
- **Corrects Muscle Imbalances**: By working each leg independently, lunges help identify and correct any strength imbalances between the left and right sides of your body. Balanced strength across both legs is essential for joint health, coordination, and even muscle development.

- **Improves Flexibility and Range of Motion**: Lunges help stretch and strengthen the hip flexors, which can become tight from prolonged sitting. Increased flexibility and range of motion in the hips make it easier to perform other exercises and prevent stiffness and discomfort.

Adding lunges to your workout routine helps build a well-rounded, functional lower body. Whether your goal is toning, weight loss, or overall strength, lunges offer benefits that enhance both your physical appearance and movement efficiency, making them an essential exercise for a strong, balanced, and fit lower body.

Basic Glute Bridge Form

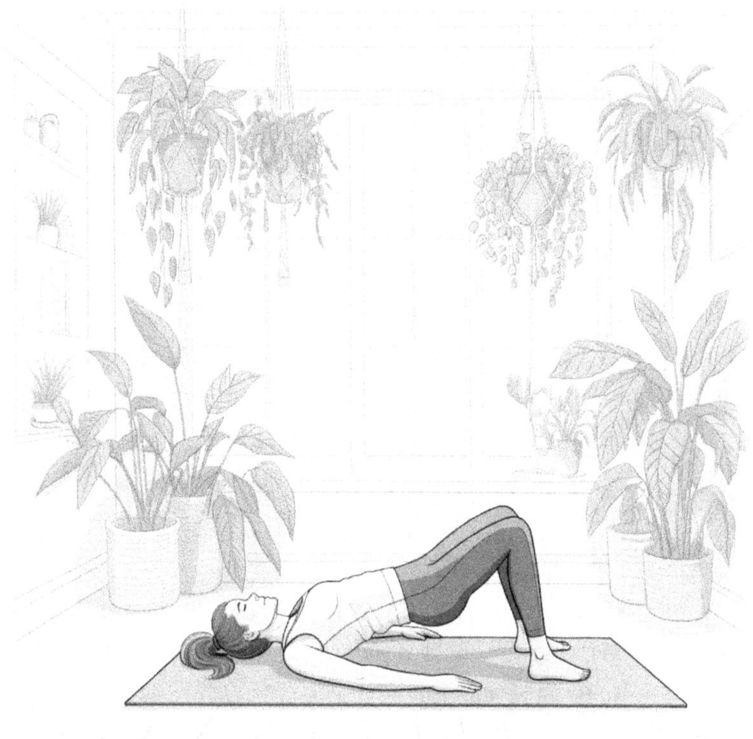

The glute bridge is a foundational exercise that effectively targets the glutes, hamstrings, and core, helping to lift and tone the backside while also strengthening the lower back. This simple yet powerful movement is perfect for beginners and advanced exercisers alike and can be done without any equipment.

Starting Position:

- Lie flat on your back with your knees bent and feet flat on the floor, hip-width apart. Your arms should rest at your sides, palms facing down.

- Position your feet so they're close enough to your glutes that you can lightly touch your heels with your fingertips.

Movement:

- Engage your core by drawing your belly button toward your spine, which will support your lower back throughout the movement.
- Press through your heels and squeeze your glutes to lift your hips toward the ceiling. Aim to create a straight line from your shoulders to your knees, making sure not to overextend your back.
- Hold the top position for a moment, squeezing your glutes and hamstrings.

Returning to Starting Position:

- Slowly lower your hips back down to the floor, maintaining control as you return to the starting position.
- Repeat for the desired number of repetitions, focusing on engaging your glutes and keeping your core tight with each lift.

The basic glute bridge is a highly effective exercise for toning and strengthening the glutes, adding lift and shape to the backside. Practicing proper form ensures that you're working the target muscles effectively, which enhances both strength and muscle tone in the lower body.

Glute Bridge Modifications for Various Fitness Levels

Glute bridges are versatile and can be adapted to suit any fitness level, making them accessible for beginners while still challenging for more advanced exercisers. Here are some modifications to help you progress safely and effectively with glute bridges:

Basic Glute Bridge Hold (Beginner):

- **How to Do It**: Perform a standard glute bridge, but hold the lifted position for a few extra seconds before lowering back down. Focus on squeezing the glutes and maintaining a stable core.
- **Benefits**: Holding the position helps beginners build glute and core strength while improving endurance in the muscles.

Single-Leg Glute Bridge (Intermediate):

- **How to Do It**: Start in the basic glute bridge position, but extend one leg straight out, keeping your thighs parallel. Press through the heel of the grounded foot and lift your hips, maintaining balance as you perform the bridge on one leg.
- **Benefits**: This variation increases the challenge for the glutes and hamstrings, as they work harder to stabilize and lift the body with only one leg. It also helps correct any muscle imbalances between the legs.

Weighted Glute Bridge (Intermediate/Advanced):

- **How to Do It**: Place a dumbbell or barbell across your hips and hold it in place as you lift into the bridge position. Make sure to maintain control and avoid overextending your lower back.
- **Benefits**: Adding weight increases resistance, making the exercise more challenging for the glutes and core. This modification is ideal for building strength and enhancing muscle definition in the lower body.

Elevated Glute Bridge (Advanced):

- **How to Do It**: Position your feet on an elevated surface, such as a bench or step, with your shoulders on the floor. Perform the bridge as usual, pressing through your heels and lifting your hips.
- **Benefits**: Elevating the feet increases the range of motion, which places more emphasis on the glutes and hamstrings and adds intensity to the movement.

Bridge Pulses (Advanced):

- **How to Do It**: In the lifted bridge position, perform small pulsing movements by lowering and lifting your hips just a few inches up and down.
- **Benefits**: Bridge pulses keep the muscles under constant tension, increasing the burn in the glutes and building muscular endurance. This variation is excellent for achieving a deeper level of muscle engagement.

These glute bridge modifications allow you to adjust the intensity of the exercise as your strength and confidence grow. By choosing the right variation, you can gradually increase the challenge, helping you build a strong, toned backside at your own pace

Benefits of Glute Bridges

Glute bridges are an incredibly effective exercise for building strength, stability, and definition in the lower body. This movement not only targets the glutes, but also engages the hamstrings and core, making it a valuable addition to any workout routine. Here's why glute bridges are so beneficial:

- **Tones and Lifts the Glutes**: Glute bridges directly target the glute muscles, helping to shape and lift the backside. Consistently incorporating this exercise can lead to a firmer, more toned appearance in the glutes, creating a lifted and sculpted look.

- **Strengthens the Hamstrings and Lower Back**: Along with the glutes, glute bridges engage the hamstrings and lower back muscles, improving overall lower body strength. This balanced development helps create a stable and supportive foundation for other exercises.

- **Enhances Core Stability**: Glute bridges require core engagement to maintain form, which helps strengthen the abdominal muscles and stabilize the lower back. This core activation contributes to improved posture and a more stable midsection.

- **Reduces Lower Back Pain**: By strengthening the glutes and core, glute bridges help alleviate stress on the lower back. Weak glutes and a lack of core stability can often lead to lower back discomfort, so building strength in these areas provides extra support for the spine.

- **Improves Hip Mobility**: Glute bridges gently stretch the hip flexors while strengthening the glutes, helping to increase hip mobility and flexibility. This benefit is especially helpful for counteracting tightness from prolonged sitting, which can affect posture and movement.

- **Boosts Athletic Performance**: Strong glutes and hamstrings are essential for explosive movements, such as jumping and sprinting. Regularly performing glute bridges can enhance athletic performance, making activities like running, cycling, and climbing stairs more powerful and efficient.

Adding glute bridges to your routine is a simple yet powerful way to tone the glutes, enhance lower body strength, and improve core stability. Whether your goals are aesthetic, functional, or a mix of both, glute bridges deliver a range of benefits that support a strong, balanced, and resilient lower body.

Basic Side Leg Lift Form

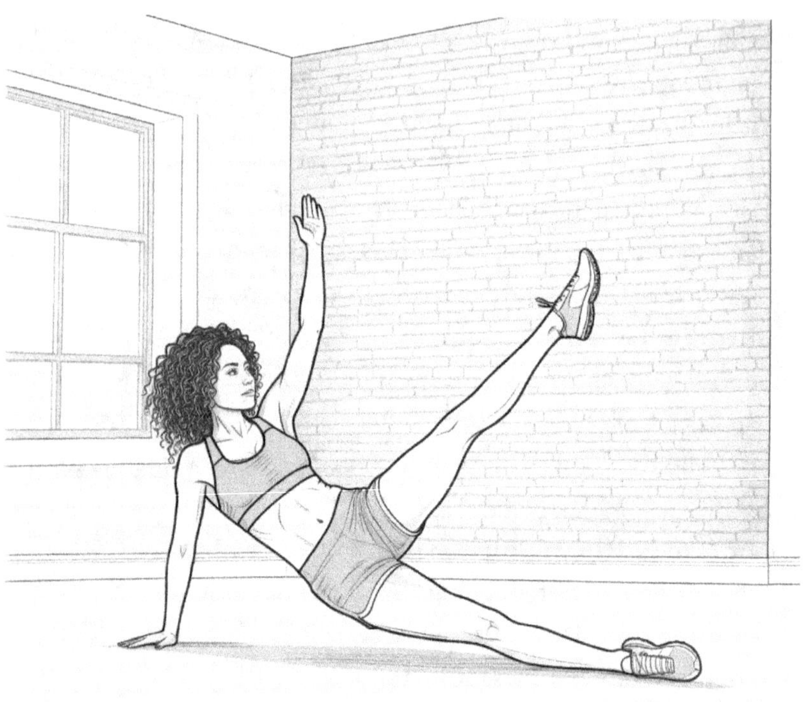

The side leg lift is a simple yet effective exercise that targets the outer thighs and glutes, helping to shape and tone the sides of the legs and hips. This move also engages the core for stability, making it a great addition to any lower body workout. Here's how to perform a basic side leg lift with proper form:

Starting Position:

- Lie on your side with your legs stacked on top of each other. Extend both legs straight, keeping your body in a straight line from head to toes.
- Rest your head on your bottom arm, or prop your head up with your hand for comfort. Place your top hand on the floor in front of you for support.

Movement:

- Keeping your top leg straight, lift it up toward the ceiling, aiming to lift it as high as comfortably possible without tilting your hips forward or backward.
- As you lift, focus on engaging the muscles in your outer thigh and glute, and keep your core tight to maintain balance.

Returning to Starting Position:

- Slowly lower your leg back down with control, keeping it straight and stacked over the bottom leg.
- Repeat for the desired number of repetitions, then switch to the other side.

The side leg lift is an excellent exercise for toning the outer thigh and glute muscles. Practicing this movement with proper form helps create definition along the hip and thigh area, adding balance and shape to your lower body.

Benefits of Side Leg Lifts

Side leg lifts are a highly effective exercise for toning and strengthening the outer thighs and glutes. This simple movement offers a range of benefits, making it a valuable addition to any workout routine focused on shaping and defining the lower body. Here's why side leg lifts are so beneficial:

- **Tones the Outer Thighs and Hips**: Side leg lifts target the muscles along the outer thigh and hip, helping to sculpt and define these areas. Consistently practicing this exercise can add shape and balance to the legs, giving them a more streamlined and toned appearance.
- **Lifts and Strengthens the Glutes**: By engaging the glutes, side leg lifts contribute to a firmer, more lifted backside. This exercise helps build the smaller, stabilizing muscles around the hips, adding overall strength and enhancing the shape of the glutes.
- **Improves Hip Stability and Balance**: Side leg lifts require core engagement and hip stability to perform correctly. This focus on balance strengthens the muscles around the hip joint, reducing the risk of injury and improving stability in other movements and exercises.
- **Supports Joint Health and Mobility**: Strengthening the outer thigh and hip muscles can help stabilize the knee joint and improve hip mobility. This benefit is especially important for reducing strain on the knees and hips, supporting healthy joint function during everyday activities.
- **Enhances Core Engagement**: Side leg lifts naturally engage the core as you work to keep your body stable throughout the movement. This extra core activation helps strengthen the abdominal muscles, improving posture and stability.

Incorporating side leg lifts into your routine is a great way to build strength and definition in the outer thighs and glutes, while also enhancing hip stability and core engagement. Whether your goal is to tone, shape, or improve balance, side leg lifts offer a range of benefits that support a strong and balanced lower body. Now that we've learned all about how to sculpt and tone our lower bodies, let's dive into some upper body exercises. In the next chapter, I'm going to share some amazing upper body sculpting exercises to get you nice and cut in no time!

Chapter 7: Upper Body Sculpting

A strong, toned upper body not only adds to a sleek, sculpted figure, but also enhances posture, functional strength, and body balance. This chapter introduces powerful exercises to help you define and shape your chest, shoulders, and arms. By focusing on moves like pushups, tricep dips, and inchworms, you'll learn foundational techniques and progressions that build lean muscle and targeted definition. Mastering these exercises will support you in creating a balanced, refined upper body that looks both fit and beautifully sculpted.

Basic Pushup Form

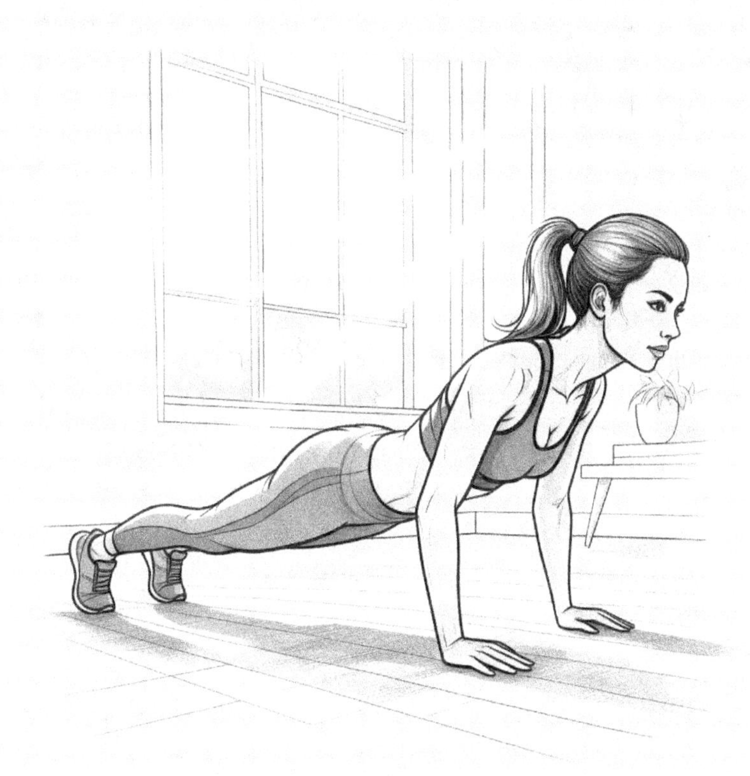

The pushup is a classic and highly effective exercise for building upper body strength, particularly in the chest, shoulders, triceps, and core. Performing a pushup with proper form ensures you're engaging the right muscles while avoiding unnecessary strain on your joints. Here's how to perform a basic pushup:

Starting Position:

- Begin in a plank position, with your hands placed slightly wider than shoulder-width apart. Your fingers should be pointing forward, and your wrists aligned directly under your shoulders.

- Keep your body in a straight line from head to heels. Engage your core by pulling your belly button toward your spine, and squeeze your glutes to maintain stability throughout the movement.

Movement:

- Slowly bend your elbows, lowering your chest toward the floor. Keep your elbows at about a 45-degree angle from your body, avoiding flaring them out too far to the sides.
- Aim to lower yourself until your chest is just above the floor, maintaining a straight line through your body. Keep your head aligned with your spine, looking slightly ahead to prevent neck strain.

Returning to Starting Position:

- Press through your palms to straighten your arms, lifting your body back to the starting plank position.
- Focus on keeping your core tight and body aligned as you push back up.

Practicing proper pushup form helps you maximize the effectiveness of the exercise by targeting the intended muscles while reducing the risk of injury. This foundational movement builds strength and definition in the upper body, making it a valuable addition to any fitness routine.

Pushup Variations

Adding variations to your pushups can help target specific muscles and keep your workout fresh and challenging. Each variation shifts the focus to different areas of the upper body, helping you achieve balanced strength and tone. Here are three effective pushup variations and the muscles they target:

Incline Pushup:

- **How to Do It**: Place your hands on an elevated surface, such as a bench, step, or even a sturdy countertop, and perform a pushup as usual.
- **Muscles Targeted**: The incline position reduces the intensity of the pushup, making it great for beginners or those looking to build strength gradually. This variation primarily targets the lower chest and shoulders while still engaging the triceps and core.

Decline Pushup:

- **How to Do It**: Position your feet on an elevated surface, such as a bench or step, and place your hands on the floor in a standard pushup position. Perform a pushup with your body angled downward.
- **Muscles Targeted**: The decline pushup is more challenging and places greater emphasis on the upper chest, shoulders, and triceps. This variation also intensifies core engagement, helping you build a strong, sculpted upper body.

Diamond Pushup:

- **How to Do It**: Place your hands close together under your chest, forming a diamond shape with your thumbs and index fingers. Perform a pushup while keeping your elbows close to your sides.
- **Muscles Targeted**: The diamond pushup places greater focus on

the triceps and inner chest muscles, helping to tone and define the back of the arms and add depth to the chest. This variation is ideal for building targeted strength and sculpting the arms.

Incorporating these pushup variations into your routine allows you to target specific areas of the upper body and progress in strength and definition. Each variation adds its own unique challenge, helping you develop a well-rounded and toned upper body.

Pushup Variations

Adding variations to your pushups can help target specific muscles and keep your workout fresh and challenging. Each variation shifts the focus to different areas of the upper body, helping you achieve balanced strength and tone. Here are three effective pushup variations and the muscles they target:

Incline Pushup:

- **How to Do It**: Place your hands on an elevated surface, such as a bench, step, or even a sturdy countertop, and perform a pushup as usual.
- **Muscles Targeted**: The incline position reduces the intensity of the pushup, making it great for beginners or those looking to build strength gradually. This variation primarily targets the lower chest and shoulders while still engaging the triceps and core.

Decline Pushup:

- **How to Do It**: Position your feet on an elevated surface, such as a bench or step, and place your hands on the floor in a standard pushup position. Perform a pushup with your body angled downward.

- **Muscles Targeted**: The decline pushup is more challenging and places greater emphasis on the upper chest, shoulders, and triceps. This variation also intensifies core engagement, helping you build a strong, sculpted upper body.

Diamond Pushup:

- **How to Do It**: Place your hands close together under your chest, forming a diamond shape with your thumbs and index fingers. Perform a pushup while keeping your elbows close to your sides.
- **Muscles Targeted**: The diamond pushup places greater focus on the triceps and inner chest muscles, helping to tone and define the back of the arms and add depth to the chest. This variation is ideal for building targeted strength and sculpting the arms.

Incorporating these pushup variations into your routine allows you to target specific areas of the upper body and progress in strength and definition. Each variation adds its own unique challenge, helping you develop a well-rounded and toned upper body.

Pushup Modifications for Various Fitness Levels

Pushups are versatile and can be adjusted to accommodate different fitness levels, making them accessible for beginners while still challenging for advanced exercisers. Here are some modifications to help you build strength progressively, no matter where you're starting:

Wall Pushup (Beginner):

- **How to Do It**: Stand facing a wall with your hands placed shoulder-width apart on the wall. Step back so your body is at a slight angle, then perform a pushup by bending your elbows and bringing your chest toward the wall. Push back to the starting position.
- **Benefits**: Wall pushups are ideal for those new to pushups or building upper body strength. This variation reduces the weight load, allowing you to focus on form and gradually strengthen your chest, shoulders, and triceps.

Knee Pushup (Beginner/Intermediate):

- **How to Do It**: Start in a regular pushup position, but keep your knees on the ground and your body in a straight line from your knees to your head. Perform a pushup by bending your elbows, lowering your chest toward the floor, and pushing back up.
- **Benefits**: Knee pushups reduce the weight load, but still target the chest, shoulders, triceps, and core. This modification is great for building strength and endurance as you work toward full pushups.

Negative Pushup (Intermediate):

- **How to Do It**: Begin in a regular pushup position. Slowly lower yourself down with control until your chest is just above the floor, then rest on the ground and reset to the starting position without the push back up.
- **Benefits**: Negative pushups focus on the lowering phase, which builds strength in the chest, shoulders, and triceps while helping you develop control. This is an excellent technique for those progressing toward full pushups.

Full Pushup (Intermediate/Advanced):

- **How to Do It**: Perform a regular pushup, keeping your body in a straight line from head to heels and lowering your chest to just above the floor before pushing back up.
- **Benefits**: The full pushup is an effective upper body exercise that builds strength and tones the chest, shoulders, arms, and core. This version engages multiple muscles, providing a well-rounded upper body workout.

Weighted Pushup (Advanced):

- **How to Do It**: Place a weight plate or wear a weighted vest for added resistance and perform a standard pushup.
- **Benefits**: Adding weight increases the intensity, challenging the chest, shoulders, and triceps even further. Weighted pushups are ideal for those who have mastered the full pushup and want to continue building strength and muscle tone.

These pushup modifications allow you to tailor the exercise to your current strength level while providing a path for progression. By gradually increasing the difficulty, you can safely build upper body strength, tone, and sculpted definition over time.

Benefits of Pushups

Pushups are a powerful exercise for sculpting a strong, toned upper body, and they offer numerous benefits that go beyond aesthetics. This foundational move engages multiple muscle groups and enhances functional strength, making it a valuable addition to any fitness routine. Here are some key benefits of pushups:

- **Builds Upper Body Strength**: Pushups primarily target the chest, shoulders, and triceps, helping you develop a lean, defined upper body. By consistently practicing pushups, you'll build the strength needed for a more sculpted, balanced figure.

- **Enhances Core Stability**: Pushups require core engagement to maintain proper alignment, which strengthens the abdominal muscles and improves core stability. This core activation supports a toned midsection while helping you maintain better posture and balance.

- **Improves Functional Strength**: Pushups mimic movements used in daily tasks, such as pushing, lifting, and carrying. Building strength through pushups makes these activities easier and reduces the risk of strain or injury in everyday life.

- **Increases Endurance**: By performing pushups regularly, you build muscular endurance in the upper body and core, allowing you to perform physical tasks for longer periods without fatigue. This increased endurance is beneficial for both fitness and day-to-day energy levels.

- **Supports Weight Loss and Toning**: Pushups engage large muscle groups and elevate your heart rate, which increases calorie burn. This exercise is effective for those aiming to support weight loss goals while toning and sculpting the arms, chest, and shoulders.

- **Requires No Equipment**: One of the greatest advantages of pushups is their accessibility. They can be done anywhere, anytime, without the need for equipment. This makes pushups a convenient option for building and maintaining strength on the go.

Incorporating pushups into your routine is a simple way to build upper body and core strength, enhance muscle tone, and improve overall fitness. Whether your goal is to develop a more defined upper body, get a great shoulder cut, increase endurance, or support functional strength, pushups offer a range of benefits that make them an essential exercise for a balanced, effective workout regimen.

Basic Tricep Dip Form

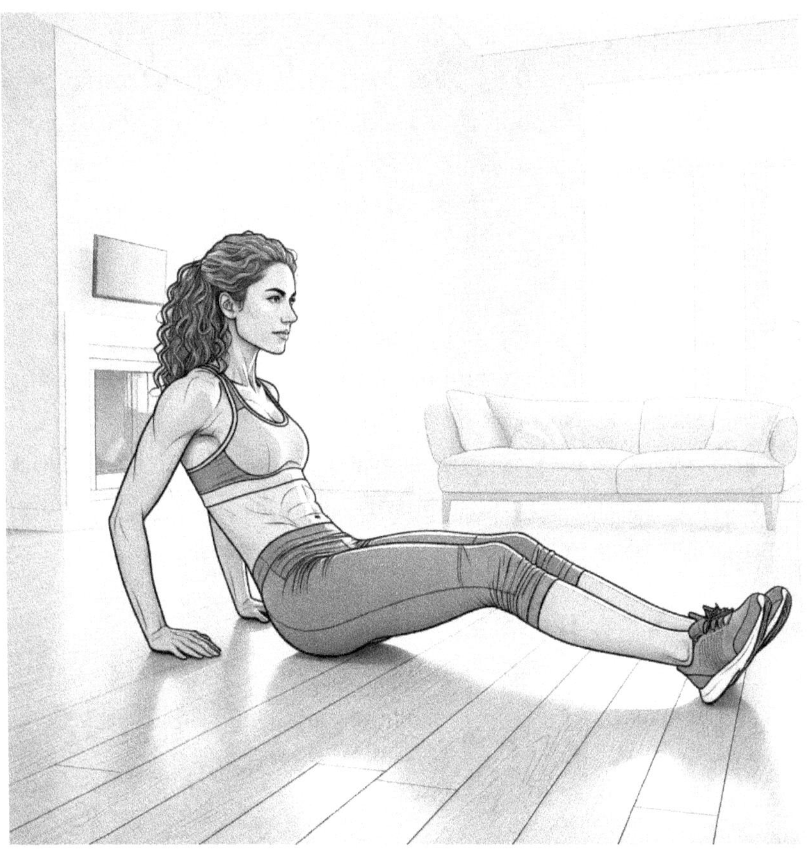

The tricep dip is an effective bodyweight exercise that targets the triceps, helping to tone and strengthen the muscles on the back of the arms (you know, that trouble area we all want to get rid of). This move also engages the shoulders and chest, making it a great addition to any upper body workout. Here's how to perform a basic tricep dip:

Starting Position:

- Sit on the edge of a sturdy surface, such as a bench, chair, or step, with your hands placed shoulder-width apart beside your hips (you can also just start on the floor), fingers facing forward.
- Slide your hips off the edge and extend your legs in front of you, keeping a slight bend in your knees for stability. Your arms should be straight, supporting your body weight.

Movement:

- Slowly bend your elbows, lowering your body down toward the floor. Keep your elbows pointing straight back, and avoid flaring them out to the sides.
- Lower yourself until your upper arms are about parallel to the floor or until you feel a comfortable stretch in the triceps. Be mindful not to go too low, as this can place strain on the shoulders.

Returning to Starting Position:

- Press through your palms to extend your arms and lift your body back up to the starting position.

Practicing proper tricep dip form ensures that you're effectively targeting the triceps and minimizing strain on the shoulders. This foundational exercise is ideal for building strength and creating a more defined, toned look in the upper arms.

Tricep Dip Modifications for Various Fitness Levels

Tricep dips can be modified to suit different fitness levels, allowing you to build strength progressively while focusing on proper form. Here are some variations to help you get the most out of tricep dips, whether you're a beginner or more advanced:

Bent-Knee Tricep Dip (Beginner):

- **How to Do It**: Sit on the edge of a sturdy surface, like a bench or chair, and place your hands beside your hips. Slide your hips off the edge with your knees bent at about a 90-degree angle and feet flat on the floor. Perform the dip movement by lowering and lifting your body.
- **Benefits**: Keeping your knees bent reduces the weight load on your arms, making the movement easier to control and ideal for beginners building tricep strength.

Feet Elevated Tricep Dip (Intermediate/Advanced):

- **How to Do It**: Place your feet on an elevated surface, such as another chair or step, while keeping your hands on the original surface. Perform the dip by bending and extending your elbows as usual.
- **Benefits**: Elevating the feet increases the load on the triceps, making the movement more challenging and allowing for greater muscle engagement in the arms, chest, and shoulders.

Weighted Tricep Dip (Advanced):

- **How to Do It**: Perform a standard tricep dip with your legs extended, but place a weight plate or dumbbell on your lap for added resistance. Keep control throughout the movement to maintain form.

- **Benefits**: Adding weight intensifies the exercise, challenging the triceps and shoulder muscles further. This variation is ideal for those who have mastered bodyweight dips and want to increase strength and muscle definition.

Assisted Tricep Dip (Beginner):

- **How to Do It**: Perform a tricep dip with your feet flat on the floor and a slight bend in your knees. Use your legs to assist by pressing lightly through your feet as you push up from the bottom of the dip.
- **Benefits**: This modification provides extra support, allowing beginners to build tricep strength and practice proper form while gradually reducing the assistance over time.

These tricep dip modifications allow you to tailor the exercise to your current strength level and make progress at your own pace. By starting with an easier variation and gradually working up to more challenging options, you can effectively build strong, defined triceps and enhance upper body endurance and stability.

Benefits of Tricep Dips

Tricep dips are a highly effective exercise for toning and sculpting the upper arms, particularly the triceps, giving your arms a sleek, defined look. This accessible bodyweight movement offers several benefits that contribute to a more sculpted and balanced upper body. Here's how tricep dips help you achieve a toned, lean figure:

- **Targets and Tones the Triceps**: Tricep dips directly engage the triceps, helping to firm and shape the back of the arms. Consistently incorporating this exercise into your routine can reduce arm flabbiness and add definition, creating a more toned, sculpted appearance.

- **Shapes the Shoulders and Chest**: Although focused on the triceps, tricep dips also work the shoulders and chest, contributing to a balanced, contoured upper body. This secondary engagement helps to create a lifted, sculpted look across the entire upper arm and shoulder area.
- **Builds Arm Endurance for a Leaner Look**: Tricep dips increase muscular endurance in the upper body, allowing you to perform more reps over time. This endurance-building effect helps tone the arms, shoulders, and chest, promoting a lean, streamlined look.
- **Supports Joint Stability for Defined Movement**: By strengthening the muscles around the elbows and shoulders, tricep dips add stability to these joints. This enhanced stability allows for controlled, precise movements, helping to accentuate and refine muscle definition.
- **Requires Minimal Equipment**: Tricep dips can be performed almost anywhere with a stable surface, making them a convenient and effective exercise for toning on the go. Whether at home or in the gym, tricep dips offer an easy way to target and sculpt the arms.

Incorporating tricep dips into your workout routine is an excellent way to sculpt the upper arms and create a toned, balanced look across the shoulders and chest. With consistent practice, tricep dips can help you achieve lean, defined arms that add to a sleek, sculpted silhouette.

Basic Inchworm Form

The inchworm is a dynamic exercise that targets the upper body, core, and hamstrings, helping to build strength, stability, and flexibility. This movement combines stretching with strength work, making it a great addition to warm-ups or as part of a full-body workout. Here's how to perform a basic inchworm:

Starting Position:

- Stand with your feet hip-width apart and your arms relaxed at your sides.
- Engage your core and keep your legs as straight as possible, but allow a slight bend in your knees if needed for comfort.

Movement:

- Bend at the hips and reach your hands toward the floor, aiming to touch the ground in front of your feet.
- Walk your hands forward, one at a time, until you reach a high plank position with your hands directly under your shoulders. Your body should form a straight line from head to heels.
- Hold the plank for a brief moment to engage your core and shoulders.

Returning to Starting Position:

- Walk your hands back toward your feet, keeping your legs as straight as possible, and return to a standing position.

The inchworm is a versatile exercise that builds upper body and core strength while stretching the hamstrings and calves. Practicing proper inchworm form helps improve flexibility, stability, and strength, making it an excellent move for overall body conditioning.

Benefits of the Inchworm

The inchworm is a multi-functional exercise that provides a range of benefits for both strength and flexibility, making it a valuable addition to any workout routine. This movement targets the upper body, core, and hamstrings while also improving mobility, balance, and coordination. Here's why the inchworm is so beneficial:

- **Strengthens the Upper Body and Core**: The inchworm engages the shoulders, chest, and arms as you walk out into a plank, helping to build strength in these areas. Holding the plank position also activates the core, promoting a stronger, more stable midsection.
- **Enhances Flexibility and Mobility**: The forward reach and walk-out in the inchworm stretch the hamstrings, calves, and lower back. This dynamic stretch improves flexibility and range of motion, especially in the hamstrings, making it an excellent warm-up or cooldown exercise.
- **Boosts Core Stability**: Holding a plank during the inchworm challenges the core, building stability and endurance. This core activation supports better posture and balance, helping you achieve a lean, toned midsection.
- **Improves Coordination and Balance**: The inchworm requires coordination between the upper and lower body as you move from standing to plank and back. This dynamic movement enhances body awareness, coordination, and balance, which can translate into improved performance in other exercises.
- **Increases Blood Flow and Warms Up Muscles**: As a full-body movement, the inchworm increases circulation and warms up the muscles, making it ideal for prepping the body for more intense workouts. It gently raises the heart rate and activates multiple muscle groups, ensuring you're ready for additional exercise.

Incorporating the inchworm into your routine helps build upper body and core strength, improve flexibility, and boost overall mobility. Whether used as a warm-up, part of a circuit, or a standalone exercise, the inchworm delivers benefits that support a balanced, well-conditioned body. No full-body workout book would be complete without providing exercises on the abs or "core". In the next chapter, I'm going to share some super ab toning exercises to blast that belly fat and get your midsection ripped! Let's get started!

Chapter 8: Core Conditioning

A strong, toned core doesn't just look amazing—it's the foundation for overall body strength, stability, and balance. This chapter focuses on exercises that target the abs, obliques, and lower belly, helping you achieve a lean, sculpted midsection. With exercises like planks, reverse crunches, bicycle crunches, and Plank Jacks, you'll work on building definition and strength in a way that supports better posture and a confident silhouette. These movements are designed to tighten and shape the core, giving you that sleek, flat stomach and adding graceful definition to your waistline.

Basic Plank Form

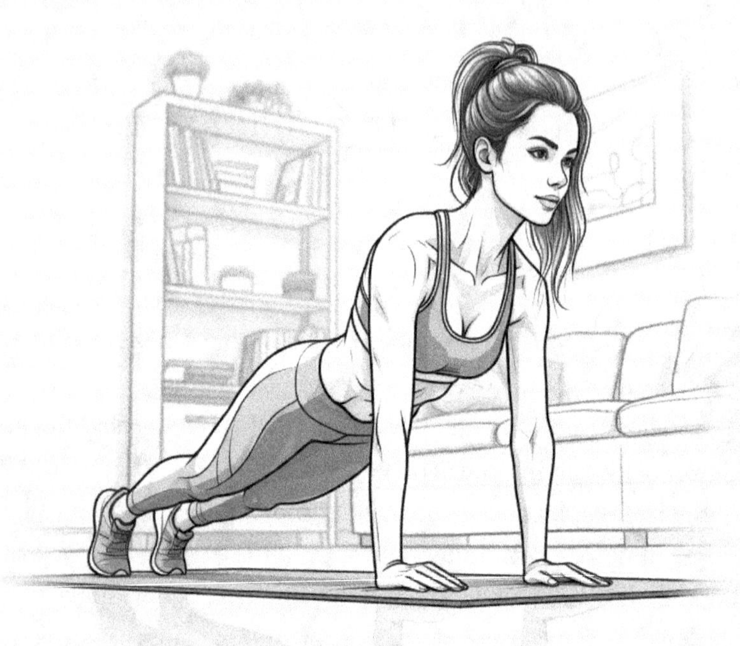

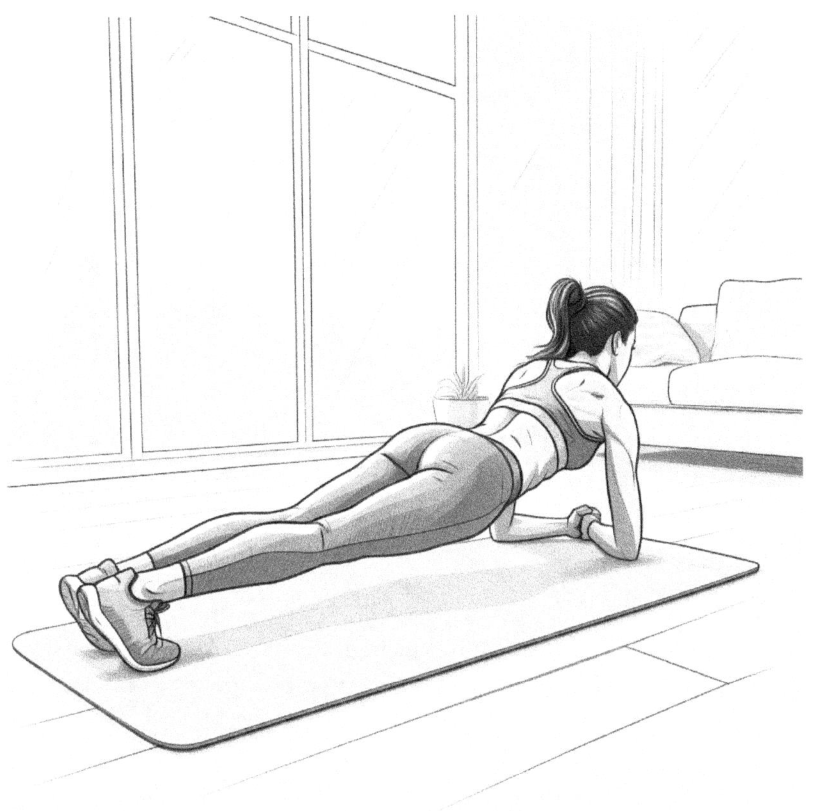

The plank is one of the most effective exercises for toning and strengthening your core, creating a sleek, defined midsection. This simple, foundational move engages multiple muscle groups and, when done with proper form, helps you build a flat, strong stomach while supporting overall body stability. Here's how to perform a basic plank:

Starting Position:

- Begin by lying face down on the floor. Place your elbows directly under your shoulders, with your forearms parallel and your palms flat on the ground.

- Extend your legs behind you, keeping your feet hip-width apart and your toes tucked under.

Movement:

- Lift your body off the ground, creating a straight line from your head to your heels. Engage your core by drawing your belly button toward your spine.
- Keep your hips level—don't let them sag or lift too high—and focus on maintaining a neutral spine by keeping your neck aligned with your back.

Hold Position:

- Hold the plank position, breathing steadily. Aim to keep your core tight and your entire body stable, avoiding any movement or swaying.

Holding a plank with proper form activates your core and engages the abdominals, helping you build strength and tone in your midsection. Practicing this foundational exercise regularly will support a firm, flat stomach and a balanced, strong core.

Plank Variations

Incorporating plank variations into your routine allows you to target different areas of the core and add variety to your workouts, keeping your core conditioning challenging and effective. Each of these plank variations brings a unique focus, helping you tone and define your midsection from multiple angles.

Side Plank:

- **How to Do It**: Lie on one side with your legs extended and stacked on top of each other. Place your elbow directly under your shoulder and lift your hips off the ground, creating a straight line from head to feet. Keep your top hand on your hip or reach it up toward the ceiling.
- **Muscles Targeted**: The side plank primarily targets the obliques, the muscles along the sides of your core, helping to slim and define the waistline. It also engages the shoulders and hips, supporting balance and stability in the upper and lower body.

Forearm Plank:

- **How to Do It**: Start in a plank position on your forearms, with your elbows directly under your shoulders and your body in a straight line from head to heels. Keep your core tight, hips level, and hold the position.
- **Muscles Targeted**: The forearm plank engages the entire core, especially the deep abdominal muscles, for a more intense core burn. It also strengthens the shoulders, arms, and glutes, making it a powerful full-body exercise that builds overall stability and endurance.

Plank Jacks:

- **How to Do It**: Begin in a high plank position with your hands directly under your shoulders. Jump your feet out wide, then jump them back together, similar to a jumping jack, but in a plank position. Keep your core tight and avoid letting your hips lift or sag.

- **Muscles Targeted**: Plank jacks target the core while adding a cardio element, making it a great exercise for toning the abs and burning calories. This variation also works the shoulders, glutes, and legs, helping to sculpt and strengthen multiple muscle groups.

By adding these plank variations to your routine, you can target specific areas of the core, boost your endurance, and keep your workouts engaging. Each variation provides a unique benefit for shaping and defining your midsection, helping you work toward a leaner, more toned core.

Plank Modifications for Various Fitness Levels

Planks are versatile and can be easily modified to suit different fitness levels, making them accessible for beginners and challenging for those with more experience. Here are some plank modifications that allow you to tailor the intensity and build core strength progressively.

Knee Plank (Beginner):

- **How to Do It**: Start in a plank position on your forearms or hands, but keep your knees on the ground rather than extending your legs fully. Maintain a straight line from your head to your knees, engaging your core.
- **Benefits**: This variation reduces the weight load on your core, making it ideal for beginners to build initial strength while practicing good form. It also reduces pressure on the lower back, helping you develop core endurance gradually.

High Plank (Beginner/Intermediate):

- **How to Do It**: Place your hands directly under your shoulders and extend your legs behind you, creating a straight line from head to heels. Keep your core tight and avoid letting your hips sag.
- **Benefits**: The high plank position engages the core, shoulders, and arms, offering a full-body challenge. It's a good next step for those comfortable with the knee plank and looking to build more upper body and core strength.

Elevated Plank (Beginner/Intermediate):

- **How to Do It**: Perform a plank with your hands or forearms on an elevated surface, like a bench or countertop. Extend your legs behind you, keeping your body in a straight line.
- **Benefits**: Elevating the plank reduces the load on the core, making it easier to hold. This modification is ideal for building strength gradually and is perfect for those who want to work on form and endurance.

Weighted Plank (Advanced):

- **How to Do It**: Once in a standard plank position, place a light weight plate or wear a weighted vest to increase resistance. Focus on maintaining proper form and stability.
- **Benefits**: Adding weight increases the challenge for the core, shoulders, and arms, making it an excellent option for those looking to intensify their plank routine and build greater strength and muscle tone.

Plank with Toe Taps (Intermediate/Advanced):

- **How to Do It**: Begin in a standard plank position and alternate tapping each foot out to the side, keeping your core stable and hips level.

- **Benefits**: This modification adds movement and engages the glutes, hips, and legs, providing a full-body challenge while intensifying core activation.

By using these plank modifications, you can tailor the exercise to your current fitness level and progress over time. Whether you're building initial core strength or aiming for a more advanced challenge, these variations allow you to safely work toward a stronger, more defined midsection.

Benefits of the Plank

The plank is an incredibly effective exercise for strengthening and toning the core, and it offers a range of additional benefits that support overall fitness and body conditioning. By engaging multiple muscle groups, the plank helps create a strong, stable foundation while sculpting and defining the midsection. Here are some key benefits of incorporating planks into your routine:

- **Strengthens the Core**: Planks target the entire core, including the rectus abdominis (the "six-pack" muscles), transverse abdominis, and obliques. This comprehensive engagement helps create a flat, toned stomach and builds the foundation for a strong, balanced core.
- **Improves Posture and Alignment**: Holding a plank requires maintaining a straight line from head to heels, which strengthens the muscles supporting the spine. This helps improve posture and body alignment, reducing the risk of slouching and back discomfort in daily activities.

- **Enhances Balance and Stability**: Planks activate the core, shoulders, and hips, which are essential for stability. Regular plank practice improves balance and control, making you feel more stable and coordinated in other exercises and everyday movements.
- **Tones the Upper Body and Glutes**: Planks work the shoulders, arms, and glutes, helping to sculpt and define these areas. This full-body engagement creates a lean, toned appearance in the upper body and helps lift and firm the glutes.
- **Reduces Lower Back Pain**: By strengthening the core and supporting muscles around the spine, planks can help reduce lower back pain. A strong core alleviates strain on the back, promoting better spinal alignment and stability.
- **Supports Functional Fitness**: Core stability is essential for virtually every movement, from lifting and bending to running and carrying. Planks build functional strength that translates into more efficient, comfortable movements in daily life, helping you feel stronger and more capable.
- **No Equipment Needed**: Planks can be done anywhere, making them a convenient and accessible exercise for building core strength and toning the body. This versatility allows you to incorporate planks into your routine without the need for any special equipment.

Incorporating planks into your fitness routine can help you achieve a stronger, leaner core, improved posture, and a more balanced body. Whether your goal is to sculpt your abs, enhance stability, or support overall fitness, planks provide versatile, impactful benefits that make them a staple in any workout.

Basic Reverse Crunch Form

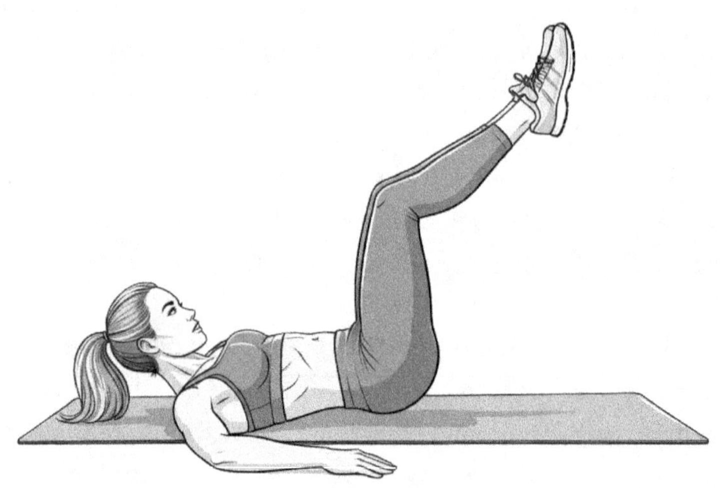

The reverse crunch is an effective core exercise that specifically targets the lower abs (the dreaded "pooch"), helping to create a flat, toned lower belly. This movement is a great addition to your core routine if you're looking to strengthen and define the lower part of your abdominal muscles. Here's how to perform a basic reverse crunch:

Starting Position:

- Lie flat on your back with your arms at your sides, palms facing down for support.
- Lift your legs, bending your knees at a 90-degree angle, so your

thighs are perpendicular to the floor and your knees are aligned over your hips.

Movement:

- Engage your core by drawing your belly button toward your spine.
- Using your lower abs, lift your hips off the floor slightly as you bring your knees toward your chest in a controlled motion. Focus on squeezing the lower abs throughout the movement.
- Avoid using momentum; instead, rely on your core strength to lift and lower.

Returning to Starting Position:

- Slowly lower your hips back down to the floor, bringing your legs back to the 90-degree angle without letting your feet touch the ground to keep tension on the abs.

Practicing the reverse crunch with proper form effectively engages the lower abs, helping to tone and flatten the lower belly. This foundational movement supports a balanced, well-defined core, making it an essential exercise for core conditioning.

Benefits of the Reverse Crunch

The reverse crunch is a go-to exercise for anyone looking to target lower belly fat, tone the core, and achieve a ripped midsection. Unlike traditional crunches, which mainly work the upper abs, the reverse crunch zeroes in on the lower abs, helping to flatten and define the lower stomach area. Here's how the reverse crunch can help you get a lean, sculpted core:

- **Targets Lower Belly Fat**: The reverse crunch effectively engages the lower abs, which can be tough to reach with standard ab exercises. By focusing on this area, the reverse crunch helps tighten and tone the lower belly, aiding in the appearance of a leaner, flatter stomach.

- **Tones and Sculpts the Midsection**: Consistent practice of reverse crunches builds strength and definition in the lower abdominal muscles, creating a balanced look across the entire core. This move helps carve out a more sculpted, ripped midsection by specifically working the lower abs.

- **Supports a Strong, Stable Core**: Building strength in the lower abs improves core stability, making your entire midsection stronger and more balanced. This enhanced stability not only supports better posture, but also helps you feel more controlled and powerful in your movements.

- **Reduces Strain on the Lower Back**: Reverse crunches, when performed correctly, are gentle on the spine and lower back. Strengthening the lower abs through reverse crunches helps alleviate pressure on the lower back, supporting a stronger, more resilient core without unnecessary strain.

- **Contributes to a Flat, Defined Stomach**: By focusing on the lower abs, the reverse crunch tightens and tones the lower belly, contributing to a flat, chiseled look. Incorporating this exercise into your routine can help achieve a ripped midsection, especially when combined with other core-focused movements.

- **No Equipment Needed**: The reverse crunch is a simple, equipment-free exercise that can be done anywhere, making it convenient to add to any workout. It's an easy way to work on your lower abs and create a toned, lean midsection without needing any special equipment.

Adding reverse crunches to your workout routine can help you work toward a toned, defined core and a flatter lower belly. This targeted move enhances your overall midsection, helping you get closer to a lean, sculpted look with consistent effort.

Basic Bicycle Crunch Form

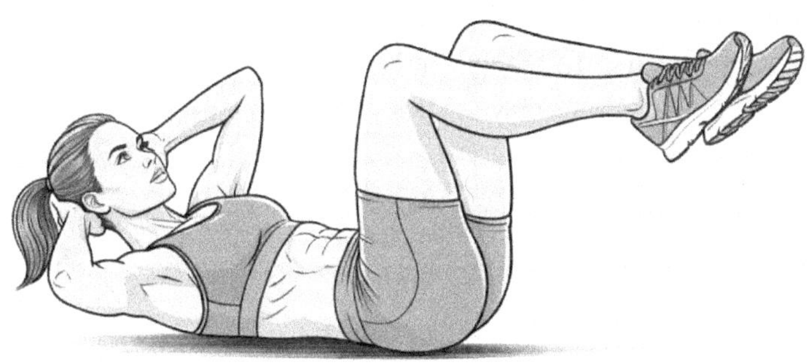

The bicycle crunch is a dynamic core exercise that targets the abs and obliques, helping to create a toned, defined waistline. This move combines core strengthening with a twisting motion to engage multiple abdominal muscles, making it highly effective for sculpting the midsection. Here's how to perform a basic bicycle crunch:

Starting Position:

- Lie flat on your back with your knees bent and feet lifted off the floor, bringing your legs into a tabletop position. Place your hands behind your head, keeping your elbows wide.
- Engage your core, pressing your lower back gently into the floor to stabilize your spine.

Movement:

- Lift your shoulder blades off the floor and bring one knee toward your chest while extending the opposite leg straight out.
- Twist your torso to bring your opposite elbow toward the knee that's bent, aiming to connect your elbow and knee as closely as possible.
- Switch sides by extending the bent leg and bringing the other knee toward your chest, twisting your torso to bring the opposite elbow toward the knee.

Continuing the Motion:

- Continue alternating sides in a controlled, cycling motion, focusing on engaging the obliques and keeping your movements steady.
- Keep your core engaged throughout, and avoid pulling on your neck by allowing the twist to come from your torso.

The bicycle crunch is an effective exercise for building core strength and toning the waist. Practicing this move with proper form helps engage both the upper and lower abs, creating a balanced, sculpted midsection and defined obliques.

Benefits of the Bicycle Crunch

The bicycle crunch is a highly effective exercise for toning and sculpting the core, with particular emphasis on the obliques and lower abs (this is one of my favorite ab exercises - it really gets the job done in a very short amount time). This dynamic movement not only builds core strength, but also helps create a lean, defined waistline. Here are the key benefits of incorporating bicycle crunches into your workout:

- **Targets the Entire Core**: The bicycle crunch engages the upper and lower abs as well as the obliques, making it a comprehensive exercise for the entire midsection. This all-around activation helps create a balanced, ripped core, enhancing both strength and appearance.
- **Defines the Waistline**: By focusing on the twisting motion, bicycle crunches effectively work the obliques, helping to shape and tone the sides of the waist. This targeted engagement is ideal for creating a more defined, contoured waistline.
- **Supports a Lean, Sculpted Midsection**: The combination of upper, lower, and side-to-side engagement in the bicycle crunch helps flatten and tone the entire core. This exercise is great for building definition and achieving a sleek, toned look across the midsection.
- **Improves Core Stability and Function**: Bicycle crunches require coordination and core control, which help strengthen the stabilizing muscles around the spine. This increased stability supports better posture and balance, making everyday movements easier and more efficient.

- **Increases Calorie Burn**: The continuous, cycling motion of the bicycle crunch adds a cardio element, which helps elevate the heart rate and increase calorie burn. This can contribute to overall fat loss, helping to reveal the toned muscles beneath.
- **No Equipment Needed**: The bicycle crunch is an equipment-free exercise that can be done anywhere, making it easy to incorporate into any routine. It's a convenient way to work on core definition and strength without the need for gym equipment.

Incorporating bicycle crunches into your routine can help you build a strong, defined core and a slimmer waistline. This exercise combines toning and calorie-burning benefits, making it an effective choice for achieving a lean, sculpted midsection. Ok, now you know the top exercises to do at home to get in amazing shape. I'm not going to stop there; however, and just leave you hanging - what kind of friend would that make me? Let's set you up for success by giving you some super simple, fast, and effective 20-minute (you heard me, just 20-minute) workouts to get you in incredible shape, toned, and losing weight.

Chapter 9: Easy 20-Minute Workouts for Visible Weight Loss, Sculpting, and Toning

These quick, effective 20-minute workouts are designed to support weight loss, toning, and body sculpting. By consistently practicing these routines, you'll boost your metabolism, burn calories, and target muscle groups to create a leaner, more sculpted silhouette. Each session combines exercises that engage different areas, helping you build strength, shape, and definition in all the right places.

Circuit Training Session 1: Lower Body Burn & Core

This session focuses on the lower body and core, combining moves to help burn calories, tone the legs, and tighten the abs.

- **Warm-Up** (4 minutes): Marching or jogging in place to elevate heart rate and activate muscles.
- **Circuit Exercises** (45 seconds each, 15 seconds rest; repeat the circuit 3 times):
- **Squats** – Tones and sculpts the thighs and glutes.

- **Reverse Crunches** – Targets the lower abs to help flatten the belly.
- **Plank Jacks** – Burns calories and engages the lower core for a lean look.
- **Lunges** – Shapes the legs and glutes, supporting overall lower body sculpting.
- **Cooldown** (4 minutes): Stretching to relax and lengthen the lower body muscles.

Total time: 20 minutes

Circuit Training Session 2: Upper Body Toning & Core

This session is all about creating toned arms, shoulders, and abs. It combines upper body and core exercises that burn calories and build lean muscle for a sculpted, defined look.

- **Warm-Up** (4 minutes): Arm circles and shoulder rolls to warm up the upper body.
- **Circuit Exercises** (45 seconds each, 15 seconds rest; repeat the circuit 3 times):
- **Push-Ups** – Engages the chest, shoulders, and arms for upper body toning.
- **Tricep Dips** – Sculpts and defines the back of the arms.
- **Bicycle Crunches** – Works the obliques and core to slim and tone the waistline.
- **Plank Hold** – Strengthens and tones the entire core for a flat, firm stomach.
- **Cooldown** (4 minutes): Stretching to release tension in the arms

and shoulders.

Total time: 20 minutes

Circuit Training Session 3: Core Shred

This intense core session is designed to burn calories and tighten the entire midsection. These moves work together to build a lean, toned core while helping you burn fat for a sculpted, flat stomach.

- **Warm-Up** (4 minutes): Light jogging or jumping jacks to activate the core and warm up the body.
- **Circuit Exercises** (45 seconds each, 15 seconds rest; repeat the circuit 3 times):
- **Plank Hold** – Builds core stability, helping create a lean, strong midsection.
- **Reverse Crunches** – Targets and tones the lower belly.
- **Bicycle Crunches** – Works the obliques to define and shape the waist.
- **Plank Jacks** – Engages the lower abs, contributing to a flatter stomach.
- **Cooldown** (4 minutes): Stretching for the abs and lower back.

Total time: 20 minutes

Circuit Training Session 4: Lower Body & Stability Sculpt

This low-impact session tones the legs, glutes, and core, helping to shape and firm the lower body without high-intensity movements. Perfect for toning and sculpting while keeping the body balanced.

- **Warm-Up** (4 minutes): Dynamic stretching for hips, legs, and core.
- **Circuit Exercises** (45 seconds each, 15 seconds rest; repeat the circuit 3 times):
- **Lunges** – Tones the thighs and lifts the glutes for a sculpted lower body.
- **Squats** – Burns calories and firms the legs and backside.
- **Plank Jacks** – Activates the lower core, helping to flatten the stomach.
- **Reverse Crunches** – Targets the lower abs, shaping a lean midsection.
- **Cooldown** (4 minutes): Stretching for the legs and hips.

Total time: 20 minutes

Circuit Training Session 5: Full Body Sculpt & Tone

This session combines calorie-burning and muscle-toning exercises to target every major muscle group. It's perfect for shedding fat and enhancing muscle definition for an all-over sculpted look.

- **Warm-Up** (4 minutes): High knees or marching in place to increase blood flow.

- **Circuit Exercises** (45 seconds each, 15 seconds rest; repeat the circuit 3 times):
- **Push-Ups** – Strengthens and defines the upper body.
- **Plank Hold** – Tones the core and creates a lean, flat stomach.
- **Bicycle Crunches** – Engages the obliques, helping to define the waist.
- **Squats** – Firms and shapes the legs and glutes.
- **Cooldown** (4 minutes): Full-body stretching to relax and lengthen muscles.

Total time: 20 minutes

Chapter 10: Bonus: 28-Day Sculpting & Toning Fitness Challenge

Welcome to your 28-Day Fitness Challenge! This program is designed to help you lose weight, tone up, and sculpt your body using the five targeted circuit training sessions. By following this plan consistently, you'll maximize calorie burn, enhance muscle definition, and achieve visible results in as little as four weeks. Each week, you'll complete a mix of the five circuits, gradually building endurance and strength while keeping your body challenged.

Weekly Structure:

- **Days 1-5**: Perform one of the circuits each day, as scheduled below.
- **Day 6**: Active recovery day (light stretching, yoga, or walking).
- **Day 7**: Rest day.

Tip: Stick to the warm-up, circuit, and cooldown for each session, focusing on form and keeping rest times consistent. Drink plenty of water and fuel your body with nutritious foods to support your progress. Minimize salt intake, as it creates water retention and excess bloating. Have fun!

Tip: For an additional calorie burn, consider adding a 20-30 minute aerobic session, such as using the elliptical, going for a run, or cycling a few days a week. This isn't necessary, and the 28-day circuit alone will give you results, this will just add a "boost" to your results.

Week 1: Building the Foundation

This week focuses on learning the exercises, building endurance, and kick starting+ weight loss.

- **Day 1**: Circuit 1 - Lower Body Burn & Core
- **Day 2**: Circuit 2 - Upper Body Toning & Core
- **Day 3**: Circuit 3 - Core Shred
- **Day 4**: Circuit 4 - Lower Body & Stability Sculpt
- **Day 5**: Circuit 5 - Full Body Sculpt & Tone
- **Day 6**: Active Recovery (30-minute walk or gentle yoga)
- **Day 7**: Rest

Week 2: Increasing Intensity

This week, we're ramping up the intensity to further support fat loss and sculpting.

- **Day 8**: Circuit 1 - Lower Body Burn & Core
- **Day 9**: Circuit 2 - Upper Body Toning & Core
- **Day 10**: Circuit 3 - Core Shred
- **Day 11**: Circuit 4 - Lower Body & Stability Sculpt
- **Day 12**: Circuit 5 - Full Body Sculpt & Tone
- **Day 13**: Active Recovery (30-minute walk or gentle yoga)
- **Day 14**: Rest

Week 3: Pushing for Progress

You'll feel stronger by now, so focus on pushing yourself a bit more each day for enhanced results.

- **Day 15**: Circuit 1 - Lower Body Burn & Core
- **Day 16**: Circuit 2 - Upper Body Toning & Core
- **Day 17**: Circuit 3 - Core Shred
- **Day 18**: Circuit 4 - Lower Body & Stability Sculpt
- **Day 19**: Circuit 5 - Full Body Sculpt & Tone
- **Day 20**: Active Recovery (30-minute walk or gentle yoga)
- **Day 21**: Rest

Week 4: Final Push

This final week is designed to maximize your efforts, helping you reach a more toned and sculpted look. Give it your best as you complete each session!

- **Day 22**: Circuit 1 - Lower Body Burn & Core
- **Day 23**: Circuit 2 - Upper Body Toning & Core
- **Day 24**: Circuit 3 - Core Shred
- **Day 25**: Circuit 4 - Lower Body & Stability Sculpt
- **Day 26**: Circuit 5 - Full Body Sculpt & Tone
- **Day 27**: Active Recovery (30-minute walk or gentle yoga)
- **Day 28**: Rest and Reflect

Tips for Success:

- **Track Your Progress**: Take "before" and "after" photos and measurements to visualize your progress.

- **Stay Hydrated**: Drinking water helps with muscle recovery and energy levels.
- **Prioritize Rest**: Ensure you get quality sleep and make the most of your rest days.
- **Focus on Form**: Quality is more important than quantity—good form ensures you get the best results and avoid injury.

Challenge Summary:

In just 28 days, this structured challenge will help you lose weight, tone up, and sculpt your entire body. With consistent effort, you'll see improvements in strength, endurance, and definition. Stick to the plan, stay motivated, and watch your body change before your eyes!

Conclusion

Congratulations on completing this journey! By following these workouts and building a routine, you've taken major steps toward achieving a more toned, sculpted, and fit body—all without needing a gym or complicated equipment. This book has equipped you with targeted exercises for weight loss, body sculpting, and toning, each designed to bring you closer to the lean, defined look you're working toward.

The journey doesn't end here; consistency is key to maintaining and building upon the progress you've made. These routines were crafted to grow with you, so revisit them, increase your intensity as you feel ready, and adjust as you get stronger. Whether your goal is to continue shedding pounds, tightening and toning, or carving out a sculpted body, you now have the tools to keep going.

Remember, the progress might feel slow at times, but every workout moves you closer to the results you want. Stick with it, stay motivated, and celebrate each small victory along the way. Fitness is not only about achieving a physical transformation, but also about boosting your confidence and strengthening your mind. The power to create a healthier, leaner, more defined body is now in your hands! But you never have to go it alone, I'm here with you, every "step" of the way!

If this book has helped you make strides toward your fitness goals, please consider leaving a review on Amazon. Your feedback can inspire others to begin their own transformation and support the creation of more resources that help people like you get fit, toned, and sculpted. Thank you for letting this guide be a part of your fitness journey. Here's to your continued success and the body you've always wanted!

References

American College of Sports Medicine. (n.d.). *ACSM's guidelines for exercise testing and prescription.* Retrieved from https://www.acsm.org

American Council on Exercise. (n.d.). *Exercise science and resources for fitness professionals.* Retrieved from https://www.acefitness.org

Centers for Disease Control and Prevention. (n.d.). *Physical activity basics.* U.S. Department of Health and Human Services. Retrieved from https://www.cdc.gov/physicalactivity/basics

International Sports Sciences Association. (n.d.). Retrieved from https://www.issaonline.com

National Academy of Sports Medicine. (n.d.). *Exercise programming and fitness guidelines.* Retrieved from https://www.nasm.org

National Academy of Sports Medicine. (n.d.). Retrieved from https://www.nasm.org

About the Author

Mia Stone is a dynamic fitness enthusiast with a deep passion for empowering others to achieve their health goals and see real results. With expertise in personal training and nutrition, Mia specializes in creating effective workout plans and motivational resources that make fitness accessible to everyone.

Her engaging writing style and practical advice focus on quick, impactful workouts and holistic wellness, all designed to help individuals achieve tangible outcomes. Mia's mission is to inspire people to embrace an active lifestyle and demonstrate that reaching fitness goals can be both enjoyable and sustainable.

Dedicated to fostering a positive mindset around fitness, Mia believes in the power of community and support. With her contagious enthusiasm and expertise, she is committed to helping others transform their lives and achieve lasting results through fitness.